THE HOME MEDIC

A First-Aid Guide For Anyone

By: Tom Nemeth

Disclaimer

The information contained in this book is intended for informational and educational purposes only and should not be construed as medical advice or a substitute for professional medical care. The author and publisher of this book make no guarantees or warranties, express or implied, regarding the accuracy, completeness, or timeliness of the information provided. It is the reader's sole responsibility to consult with a qualified healthcare professional for any and all medical needs and concerns.

Specifically, please note:

- This book is not intended as a comprehensive first-aid manual and does not cover all possible emergency situations.
- Readers should seek professional medical guidance before attempting any first-aid techniques.
- The author and publisher disclaim all liability for any injury or harm resulting from the use or misuse of the information contained in this book.
- Readers should always follow the instructions provided by emergency medical personnel in any actual

emergency.

By using this book, you agree to hold the author and publisher harmless from any and all claims, damages, or losses incurred in connection with the use of the information provided.

Additional Recommendations:

- We encourage readers to take a certified first-aid and CPR course for hands-on training and skills development.
- Keep a first-aid kit stocked with essential supplies readily available.
- Familiarize yourself with emergency contact information and procedures in your area.

We hope this book empowers you to be prepared for emergencies, but always remember that seeking professional medical assistance is crucial for ensuring the best possible outcome in any critical situation.

Images were provided by Canva ® under license use. These images can not be reproduced or sold without permission from Canva—all rights reserved with the content of the book and information/photos contained.

This product cannot be reproduced, sold, or altered in any way without permission from the seller and author.

TABLE OF CONTENTS

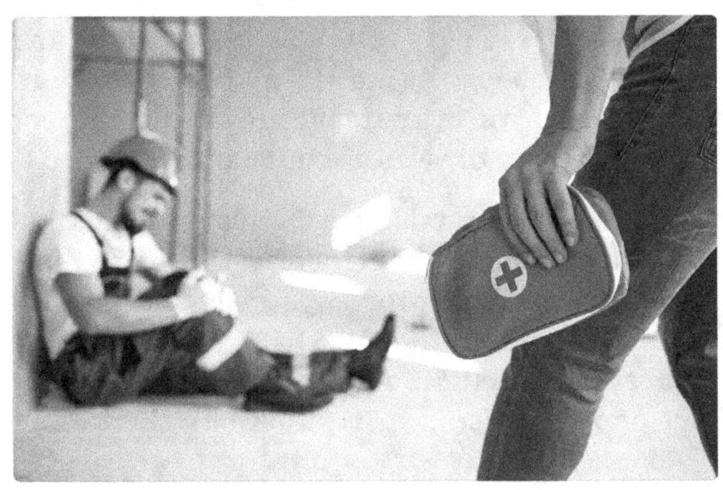

PREFACE:

Throughout our lives, unexpected events frequently arise when we least expect them to. Knowing how to give emergency care can make all the difference, from minor incidents to more significant catastrophes. The idea behind this book, "Home First Aid: A Practical Guide to Emergency Care," is a deep conviction that every home should be prepared to act efficiently when disaster strikes.

"Preparation is the key to success," as the saying goes, and this is especially true when it comes to health and safety issues. This tutorial aims to provide you with practical, simple-to-follow instructions that you can use in the convenience of your own home. We've created a thorough booklet that covers a wide range of eventualities, from simple cuts and bruises to more complicated emergencies, by drawing on current first aid standards and proven medical practices.

To assist you in navigating through various circumstances, these pages contain clear and easy-to-follow instructions and concise explanations. This book is meant to serve as your reliable companion, whether you're a parent, caregiver, or someone trying to be more ready for unforeseen circumstances.

Recall that the basis for taking effective action is knowledge. You're making a big start in the right direction by reading through the contents of this book to protect yourself and your loved ones. It's crucial to understand, though, that this book can substitute neither professional medical advice nor treatment. Always seek out prompt expert assistance in situations that are critical or potentially fatal.

Now that you have this book in your possession, you will have no trouble developing into a more competent and self-assured first responder in your own house. I hope it is a valuable tool that provides consolation and direction when needed.

I hope the voyage ahead is safe and healthy for you and your loved ones.

CHAPTER 1: INTRODUCTION TO FIRST AID

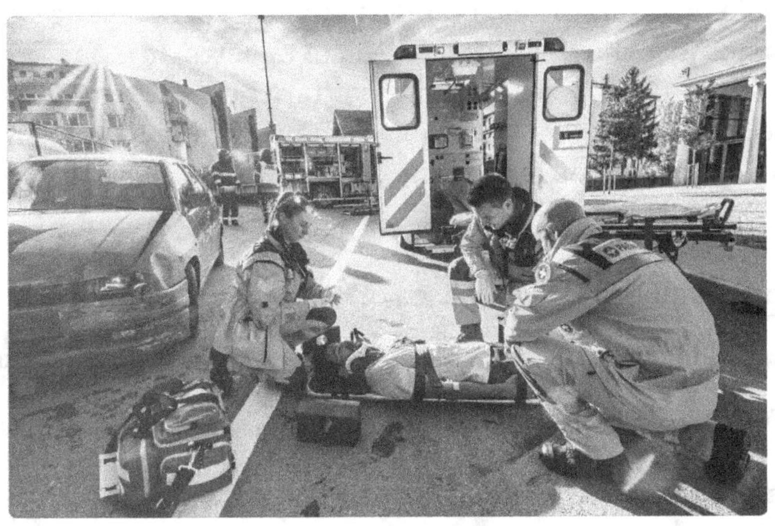

Emergencies are the unanticipated threads that lace our everyday lives together, like a tapestry in life. They can take many forms, such as a hot stove burn, a scraped knee, an unexpected chest discomfort, or a loved one choking on food. These situations call for quick response, and during these critical times, first aid training shines as a ray of hope and comfort.

First Aid's Vital Significance

Imagine a society where everyone, regardless of age or

background, has the skills and self-assurance necessary to handle situations effectively. Communities would be strengthened, pain lessened, and lives would be spared. Adopting first aid gets us one step closer to this planet.

In the stark reality of the American landscape, accidental deaths continue to hold the tragic distinction of being the leading cause of death for individuals aged 1 to 44, according to the Centers for Disease Control and Prevention (CDC). This chilling statistic underscores the ever-present vulnerability of life in its prime, a harsh reminder that unexpected dangers lurk even amidst routine activities.

First aid is a skill set that should be included in everyone's toolbox and is not just the domain of medical experts. It is the first vital treatment a patient receives right after they are hurt or become ill. We fill the gap between a crisis and expert medical care by providing timely and suitable support.

First Aid's Foundational Ideas

Fundamentally, first aid is based on three fundamental principles:

1. Save Lives: Preserving life is the primary goal of first aid.

In any emergency situation, the immediate focus should be on ensuring the person's vital functions are sustained. This involves assessing and addressing the ABCs: Airway, Breathing, and Circulation.

- **Airway**: Ensuring the person's airway is clear and unobstructed is crucial. If needed, gently tilt the head back to open the airway.
- **Breathing**: Observe for chest rise and fall, listen for breath sounds, and feel for airflow. If the person is not breathing, initiate rescue breathing or CPR as necessary.
- **Circulation**: Checking for a pulse and signs of blood circulation is essential. If there's no pulse, immediate CPR is initiated to maintain blood flow.

2. Avoid Additional Injury: The goal of first aid is to prevent the condition from worsening.

Once the primary assessment is complete and any life-threatening issues have been addressed, it's essential to take steps to prevent further harm.

- **Immobilization**: In cases of suspected fractures or spinal injuries, immobilizing the affected area helps prevent additional damage.
- **Securing the Environment**: Creating a safe environment is crucial. This may involve removing hazards, such as sharp objects or dangerous substances.
- **Stabilizing the Patient**: Ensuring the person is in a comfortable and secure position, particularly for those with injuries or medical conditions, helps prevent further harm.

3. Promote Recovery: The goal of first aid is to help the patient recover as much as possible.

After the immediate life-threatening concerns have been addressed, the focus shifts to promoting the best possible recovery for the individual.

- **Stopping Bleeding**: Applying pressure and using bandages or dressings to control bleeding is crucial in preventing further blood loss.
- **Pain Relief**: Administering appropriate pain relief measures, such as over-the-counter medications or positioning for comfort, helps ease discomfort.
- **Emotional Support**: Providing reassurance, comfort, and emotional support is vital for the well-being and mental recovery of the individual.

By adhering to these three fundamental principles, first aid providers are equipped to respond effectively to a wide range of emergencies. These principles serve as a foundation for the immediate care that can make a crucial difference in the outcome of an emergency situation. Remember, while first aid is a valuable skill, professional medical assistance should always be sought in serious or life-threatening situations.

A First Aider's Role

A first responder serves as a calming light during a crisis. They have the know-how, abilities, and self-assurance to move forward and offer aid immediately. Being present when it matters most is a luxury as much as a responsibility.

We will explore a variety of circumstances in this book, giving you the tools you need to react appropriately. You will obtain a thorough understanding of first aid, covering everything from the fundamental methods of evaluating a casualty to the more sophisticated abilities needed for particular circumstances.

Keep in mind that every little thing you do can have a significant impact as you set out on this adventure. You have the ability to save the lives of people who are in need.

We will cover a wide range of typical crises in the upcoming chapters and walk you through how to administer care immediately. By the end of this book, You will have the confidence to use first aid and a practical understanding of it.

Knowing Your Limits: The Hero's Wisdom in First Aid

The urge to help in an emergency is commendable, but true heroism lies in understanding your own capabilities and knowing when to step back. The most impactful action you can take is often not just about your skills, but about making informed decisions within the constraints of your limitations.

Safety First: Assessing the Scene Before Diving In

Before rushing into an emergency, take a moment to assess the situation. Ask yourself:

- **Is the scene safe for you and the casualty?** Fire, explosions, falling debris, or hazardous materials require immediate evacuation. Ensure your own safety before attempting to help others.
- **Can you identify the type of emergency?** Knowing if it's a bleeding wound, choking incident, or potential poisoning informs your initial response.

Honesty is Heroism: Recognizing Your Skill Level

Overestimating your abilities can be detrimental in an emergency. Be honest with yourself about your training and experience. Ask yourself:

- **Have I received proper first-aid training for this specific situation?** Performing unfamiliar techniques can worsen the situation.
- **Am I confident in my ability to remain calm and make clear decisions under pressure?** Panic and confusion can hinder effective first aid.

Stepping Aside Gracefully: When to Hand Over the Baton

Knowing when to call for help is not a sign of weakness, but a mark of wise judgment. Don't hesitate to seek professional assistance if:

- **The injury is severe or life-threatening.** Extensive bleeding, unconsciousness, or suspected spinal injuries require immediate medical attention.
- **You are unsure about the nature of the emergency.** Poisoning, allergic reactions, or complex wounds require professional diagnosis and treatment.
- **You feel overwhelmed or out of your depth.** Your own well-being is crucial. Don't hesitate to call for help if the situation feels beyond your capabilities.

Remember, reaching out for help is not a failure, but a responsible act that ensures the best possible outcome for the

casualty.

Beyond Bandages: The Power of Calling for Help

Your role as a first-aider extends beyond administering physical assistance. You are also a crucial link in the emergency response chain:

- **Provide accurate information to emergency services.** Clearly describe the situation, location, and nature of the injury.
- **Keep the casualty calm and reassured.** Your presence and support can significantly help manage pain and anxiety.
- **Follow instructions from medical professionals.** Once help arrives, assist as directed and be prepared to provide any relevant information about the initial situation.

Knowing your limits in first aid doesn't make you less of a hero. It makes you a more responsible and impactful one. By prioritizing safety, recognizing your skills, and calling for help when needed, you ensure that your courage and initiative translate into the best possible outcome for everyone involved.

Remember, true heroism lies not only in acting but also in acting wisely. This chapter equips you with the knowledge and confidence to navigate the complex landscape of first aid, allowing you to be a capable and responsible first responder within the boundaries of your abilities.

CHAPTER 2: FIRST AID ESSENTIALS

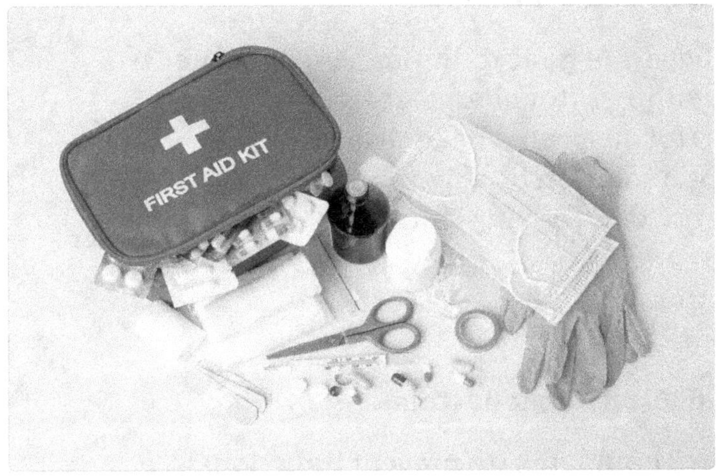

In the first aid field, readiness is crucial. A fully supplied first aid kit functions as your armory prepared to handle a range of circumstances. Having the appropriate equipment and materials on hand can be crucial in treating minor injuries such as cuts, sprained ankles, and unexpected fevers.

Putting Together a First Aid Kit

A well-stocked first aid bag is like having a reliable friend beside you whenever you need them. The following is an exhaustive inventory of necessary materials that need to be included in your kit:

Clothes and Bandages

- Adhesive bandages (various sizes)
- Rolls and pads of sterile gauze
- Adhesive tape
- Triangle bandages (used for wraps and slings)
- Elastic bandages (for sprains and strains)
- Sterile eye pads
- Sterile non-adherent dressings

Medications and Ointments

- Pain relievers (e.g., acetaminophen, ibuprofen)
- Antihistamines (for allergic reactions)
- Aspirin (for suspected heart attack)
- Antiseptic solution or wipes
- Tweezers (for removing splinters)
- Scissors
- Digital thermometer
- Tweezers

Tools and Miscellaneous Items

- Gloves without latex (to prevent infections)
- CPR face shield or mask
- Safety pins
- Flashlight with extra batteries
- Instant cold packs
- Emergency blanket - Prescription medications (if applicable)
- List of emergency numbers and contacts

In considering first aid kit costs, it's essential to recognize that prices vary based on factors like kit size, contents, and intended use. Basic kits, covering essentials like bandages and antiseptics, range from $10 to $30, while intermediate kits with a broader selection of supplies can cost between $30 and $60. Specialized or advanced kits, tailored for specific purposes, range from $60 to several hundred dollars. Home kits, designed for common injuries, fall within the intermediate range. Travel or car kits, compact for mobility, range from $10 to $50.

Professional or medical facility kits, comprehensive and designed for specific settings, can range from several hundred to thousands of dollars. Ultimately, prioritizing a well-equipped kit that aligns with your needs is paramount, whether purchasing pre-made kits or assembling custom ones. However, especially if you have small children and a large family, you should always take advantage of this step of making sure you have selected a sufficient-sized first aid kit.

Frequent Inspection and Restocking

A first aid kit is a dynamic resource that needs ongoing maintenance rather than a one-time purchase. Ensure to periodically inspect the contents for missing supplies, damaged packing, or expired materials. To ensure your kit stays prepared for any eventuality, restock and replace as necessary.

Also, items expire inside your kit and should be tracked for usable dates. These dates are crucial to regularly maintain and rotate stock to ensure expired materials are not being used that could either fail or cause additional harm during a time of need. I suggest writing expiration dates big and clear on the front of the case (if a premade or disposable case) to identify when the usable life of the kit is straightforward.

Tailor to Particular Needs

When assembling a first aid kit, it's crucial to consider the specific requirements of your household members. Consider anyone who may have specific medical needs or allergies, and make sure they have the supplies or medicines they require. This guarantees that in the event of an emergency, you will be ready to handle their particular health difficulties.

Additionally, it's critical to choose appropriate goods for the size and age of your young children if you have any. Supplies like kid-friendly thermometers, pediatric prescriptions, and child-sized bandages should all be included in your box. The kit's ability to protect children's well-being increases when its contents are modified to meet their needs.

By customizing your first aid kit to the specific requirements of your household, you're not only demonstrating a commitment to their safety but also ensuring that you're equipped to provide the best possible care in times of need. Remember, preparedness tailored to individual needs is the cornerstone of effective first aid.

Recognize Your Equipment

It is crucial that you are familiar with the items in your first aid kit. Knowing each item's function and use will enable you to react to emergencies with poise and efficiency. Being proficient with tools, bandaging procedures, and medicine administration will significantly increase your confidence and effectiveness when doing first aid.

It is important to take the time to become familiar with the contents of your first aid kit because each one is different and designed to meet the particular needs of your household. Make a note of each item's functionality and, if you can, practice using them. This practical experience guarantees that you'll be ready to use the resources available to you when the time comes.

Furthermore, it is equally vital to frequently examine and refresh your understanding of the kit's contents, as the household's demands may change over time. Frequent practice and familiarity with your first aid supplies lay the groundwork for an efficient emergency response, which in turn improves your loved one's safety and well-being.

Availability and Holding

The effectiveness of a well-stocked first aid kit depends on how convenient it is to use. Select a visible and accessible area of your house to keep your goods. Make sure it's a location that all family members can easily find in an emergency.

Everyone in your home needs to be aware of the location of the first aid kit. Remind family members—especially kids—of its position on a regular basis to help them understand how important it is to have quick access in case of emergency. You may also organize a scavenger hunt for emergency supplies to assist the kids in learning the locations of important supplies. This can contain things like first aid kits, medicine cabinets, fire extinguishers, and hazardous products like pesticides, home cleaners, and combustible materials. It can also include other dangerous items like knives, heavy objects, electrical dangers, and firearms if they are kept in the house.

Once more, everything that could endanger the family homestead should be secured away and kept out of the reach of family members. Accidental injuries remain the primary cause of death for young children, even as the CDC continues to collaborate with regional health departments and agencies. It is imperative for parents to exercise vigilance in ensuring that any materials that may present a risk to their younger family members are securely stored and inaccessible to unauthorized individuals. This is especially true with firearms and other weaponary. Always make sure weapons are unloaded, locked, and stored away to avoid accidental injuries.

Ensure your first aid items are kept in a strong, airtight container to extend their useful life. By protecting the contents from moisture, this makes sure they stay in top shape and are ready for use.

Putting together a thorough first aid pack is a great way to show off your proactive attitude toward disaster preparedness while also demonstrating your dedication to your loved ones' safety and well-being. We will go into great detail in the upcoming chapters regarding how to apply these resources to different scenarios.

Emergency Numbers

Quick access to expert assistance is essential to providing practical aid in the emergency response situation. This chapter goes over the critical actions you must take to make sure you have your most important contact information on hand when you need it most. Make a complete list of emergency phone numbers that include:

- Local emergency services, such as 911, in the United States.
- The Poison Control Center.
- Your primary care physician.
- Nearby hospitals and medical facilities.
- Specialized emergency services tailored to your unique circumstances.

Decide where in your house you want this list to be easily visible. For extra protection, think about laminating it or using a waterproof cover.

Digitize these numbers and store them in your mobile device's contacts section with clear labels. Ensure everyone in the family, especially the kids, knows how to access and use this priceless resource. Review and update this list regularly. Check to see if all the numbers are still correct and up to date, taking into account any changes to your contacts.

Include contacts for relevant specialists or support services for households with unique circumstances or specific medical needs. Make sure everyone in the family understands the importance of having these emergency contacts, starting from the youngest. Practice exercises where they might need to apply this vital knowledge. Look into smartphone apps that provide quick access to vital information and emergency services. These apps are beneficial allies during emergencies.

Ensure your household's safety and well-being are proactively protected by keeping emergency numbers readily available. Easy access to expert assistance becomes essential for a prompt and efficient response in an emergency.

CHAPTER 3: EVALUATING EMERGENCIES AND TAKING ACTION

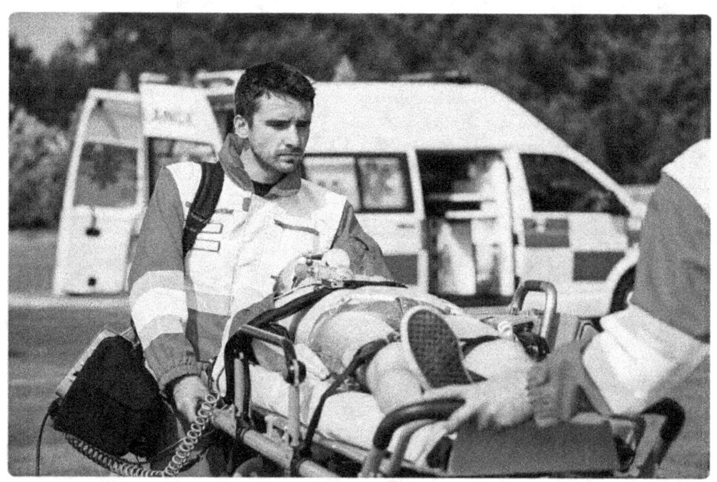

One of the most effective allies in an emergency is a calm, collected approach. This chapter gives you the tools you need to evaluate the situation correctly, estimate the extent of an injury or illness, and respond quickly.

Staying calm and collected is going to be the hardest part of your journey, when it comes to providing first aid. This triples when it comes to a family member or friend, and may even be responsible for their well-being and care. Understand that it is okay to be nervous, excited, or scared when a medical emergency happens. However, practicing and remembering how to react in the event or occurrence of an emergency will make sure it is a smooth process for you and the person in need.

The first step to have in your arsenal is understanding the basic ABCs of medical evaluation. That is *Airway, Breathing, and Circulation.* However, we are going to expand on these ideas so that you are not fixated or narrowed in your initial assessment.

Airway

A clear airway is the first step to making sure a person is safe. Without oxygen, we have no way to maintain or sustain life. The primary reason for death is a lack of oxygen to the vital organs, primarily the brain and heart. It is imperative to ensure a clear airway, if possible, is free and clear of obstructions. Your first step is to verify that there are no obstructions in the airway. To clear the airway, tilt the head back a little and visualize no obstructions. A finger sweep can be done in the event an obstruction is visualized. However, don't lose any digits (that's your fingers) in the process of removing the obstructions. We will continue more on obstructed airways in the choking section of this book.

Breathing

As we stated, lack of oxygen to the vital organs is the primary reason for death. After checking for a clear airway, your second step is to verify that the chest is moving (rising and falling) and indicate the person in front of you is breathing. Without chest movement, the lungs cannot do their primary function of getting oxygen into the bloodstream and pulling carbon dioxide (chemical waste in the blood) out of the body.

How we breathe is a highly complex process and involves several organs working in harmony. The body's respiratory system keeps the system in check to a very small window. Any deviation from this window can significantly impact the functions of our body. Within minutes of not breathing, we can have significant bodily harm that can last a lifetime. However, there are certain features that are important to know. The diaphragm is the main muscle that helps us breathe. As the diaphragm pulls down, the negative pressure causes the lungs (we have two) to pull open. The exhalation process is passive, and the stretching of the rib cage helps pull the chest back to its relaxed position. As we breathe in, we are pulling oxygen in the air. As we exhale, we are disposing of carbon dioxide that builds in the blood as we create waste and energy in the body.

Now that you know why and how we breathe, let's discuss what you should look for.

- Always look for chest rise and fall in a person.
- Adults breath at 12-20 breaths per minute. Children are anywhere from 18-25/30, depending on age. Babies typically breathe from 30-50 breaths per minute.
- Pay attention and feel warm air or breath coming from the individual.
- Start mechanical breaths if the person isn't breathing but has a pulse. If there isn't a pulse, then that's when we talk about circulation.

Circulation

Even though circulation is third, it definitely doesn't separate its importance from the other two. Without the heart circulating oxygen-rich blood with nutrients to the organs, we could not survive. The heart is an amazing organ that has been evolutionary designed to keep going through some of the harshest conditions imaginable. It has several unique features, including automaticity (self-regulation in the absence of the brain), specialized branched muscle fibers that don't fatigue like your skeletal muscles, and separate chambers to help keep the oxygenated blood and deoxygenated blood separate from each other.

Without continuous circulation, several physiological conditions happen. Carbon dioxide will build up in the blood, which causes the blood to become acidic. The body requires a precise acid/base balance to complete many tasks. The process of the body becoming acidic can happen very quickly, causing many organs to become damaged or lose functionality.

Secondly, the body uses the blood transportation system to filter the blood of used components and toxins. The body has many filters, such as your Liver, Spleen, and Kidneys. Without the blood being able to filter through these vital organs, many chemicals and waste will continue to build and have no way of clearing.

Thirdly, your circulatory system delivers oxygen and removes carbon dioxide (CO_2 - from dioxide, meaning two oxygens to one carbon) from every square inch of your body. Oxygen is the life force that we use to create energy in our cells. We have specialized cells called red blood cells that have been designed to attract both Oxygen and CO_2.

- Check for a pulse (carotid or radial). The human heart beats typically at 60-100 for adults, 60-120 for children, and 100-160 for babies (these ranges vary per age, so make sure to talk with your pediatrician about what is suitable for your child).
-Check for a pulse on the carotid artery or wrist for at least 5 seconds but no more than 10 seconds.
- If absent, initiate CPR (we will cover this subject in a later chapter)

Disability

In emergencies, it's important to remember that individuals with disabilities may require special attention and accommodations. By being prepared and knowledgeable, you can provide adequate first-aid support to people with disabilities. This segment will cover critical considerations and techniques to ensure their safety and well-being during emergencies.

Disabilities can vary significantly in terms of type and severity. Some common disabilities include mobility impairments, visual or hearing impairments, intellectual or developmental disabilities, and mental health conditions. It's essential to approach each situation with empathy, respect, and patience while considering the specific needs of the person you are assisting.

Communication: Effective communication is crucial when providing first aid to individuals with disabilities. Remember to speak clearly and calmly, using simple language. If the person has a hearing impairment, consider using written or visual communication aids. For those with speech impairments, encourage them to communicate through alternative methods, such as using gestures or pointing to relevant body parts.

Mobility and Evacuation: When assisting someone with a mobility impairment, be aware of their specific needs. Check if they use any mobility aids, such as a wheelchair or crutches, and ensure they are accessible during the emergency. If evacuation is necessary, offer assistance, but always ask for their preferred method of help. Avoid moving individuals with potential spinal injuries unless there is an immediate threat to their safety.

Visual and Hearing Impairments: For individuals with visual impairments, describe any actions or procedures you are performing and ask for their consent before assisting. If they have a guide dog, ensure it remains with the person during the emergency. Similarly, when attending to someone with a hearing impairment, try to establish visual contact and consider using written communication or sign language if possible.

Intellectual or Developmental Disabilities: When aiding someone with an intellectual or developmental disability, it's crucial to maintain a calm and patient demeanor. Provide clear instructions and allow them enough time to process and respond. Be mindful of sensory sensitivities and adapt your approach accordingly. If necessary, seek assistance from caregivers or family members who may be familiar with the individual's specific needs and communication style.

Mental Health Conditions: During emergencies, individuals with mental health conditions may experience heightened anxiety or distress. Approach them calmly and offer reassurance. Avoid making assumptions or judgments about their condition. If the person is experiencing a crisis or suicidal ideation, prioritize their safety and seek professional help immediately.

By understanding and considering the specific needs of individuals with disabilities, you can ensure that your first aid response is inclusive and effective. Remember to communicate clearly, adapt your techniques when necessary, and always treat every person with dignity and respect.

Exposure

When it comes to exposure in the context of dignity, it typically refers to the act of revealing or sharing personal information, experiences, or vulnerabilities. It is important to approach this topic with sensitivity and respect for the individual's autonomy and privacy. Emergency situations can be raw and vulnerable, putting people in very uncomfortable situations. There are many things to consider when in a first-aid situation.

Respect Confidentiality: Recognize that personal information should be treated with utmost confidentiality. Only share information with appropriate individuals who have a legitimate need to know. Maintaining confidentiality helps preserve a person's privacy and allows them to control the narrative of their own experiences.

Seek Informed Consent: When discussing personal stories or experiences, always seek consent from the individual before sharing or exposing any details. Allow them to decide what information they are comfortable sharing and ensure they understand the potential impact of their disclosure.

Create a Safe and Non-judgmental Environment: Foster an atmosphere of trust and acceptance where individuals feel comfortable sharing their experiences without fear of judgment or stigma. Encourage open communication and actively listen to their concerns or stories, providing support and empathy.

Empower Autonomy: Recognize and respect an individual's right to choose how much of their personal information they wish to expose. Avoid pressuring or coercing them into revealing more than they are comfortable with. Allow them to set their boundaries and determine the pace at which they share their experiences.

Provide Resources and Support: Offer information about available resources, such as support groups, counseling services, or helplines, that can assist individuals in addressing their concerns or finding further assistance. Empowering them with knowledge and options can help them make informed decisions about exposure and accessing support.

Remember, each individual's experiences and choices regarding exposure are unique, and it is essential to approach the topic with sensitivity, respect, and a focus on supporting their dignity throughout the process. Sometimes, this isn't always possible (the person is unconscious or in a public place), but we should always limit an individual's exposure and protect their dignity.

Dialing for Help

In this stage you may have recognized the person is exhibiting a life-threatening emergency. At this time, it's imperative that we dial for help so we can facilitate emergency care. Many life-saving techniques you will learn in this book will be for nothing if emergency services are never contacted. As soon as an emergency is recognized, it's important to remember that either you or a designee is instructed to contact emergency services

Immediately. Time is of the essence in these scenarios, so always remember this crucial step.

If you need immediate assistance or support, I highly recommend dialing emergency services in your country. The emergency number can vary depending on where you are located. In many countries (for us in the United States), the emergency number is 911, but it may differ in your region.

Emergency services are equipped to handle urgent situations and can provide the necessary help you need. Depending on the nature of the emergency, they can dispatch medical professionals, law enforcement, or other appropriate support.

If you are not facing an immediate emergency but still require assistance, consider contacting helplines or hotlines specializing in the specific issue you are dealing with. There are helplines available for a wide range of concerns, such as mental health, domestic violence, substance abuse, and more. These helplines are staffed by trained professionals who can provide guidance, support, and connect you with additional resources if needed.

It's important to remember that seeking help is a sign of strength, and there are people out there who are ready and willing to assist you.

Secondary Evaluation

After the initial assessment is finished and any potentially fatal problems have been resolved, go on to a more thorough assessment of the patient's state. At this stage in the evaluation, you should have a clear understanding of what you are dealing with. This will give you time to make informed decisions and have a clear avenue in assessing the victim's status. This entails performing a head-to-toe examination for any injuries or disease-related symptoms. It's important to understand that even though the following conditions may not fall under the initial evaluation, they could still require emergency services or immediate treatment. It's your job as the first responder to make sure appropriate action is taken.

Non-Critical Conditions

- In less severe situations, consult a physician or go to a hospital.

Bleeding

Bleeding, whether from a minor cut or a more serious injury, requires prompt attention and appropriate care. This section will guide you through the steps to control and treat bleeding effectively. We will provide more information in this section and a later chapter, but it's imperative to have a quick refresher on typical bleeding situations.

Start by assessing the severity of the bleeding. Determine if it is minor or requires immediate medical attention. Remember, severe bleeding or bleeding that doesn't stop may indicate a more serious injury and should be addressed promptly by medical professionals.

For minor bleeding, apply direct pressure to the wound using a clean cloth or gauze pad. Maintain firm pressure for several minutes to encourage clotting and control the bleeding. Elevate the affected body part greater than the level of the heart to help reduce blood flow.

Once the bleeding is under control, gently cleanse the wound with mild soap and water. You may also use sterile saline if you have this readily available. This step helps minimize the risk of infection. Avoid using harsh chemicals or alcohol directly on the wound, as they can cause further damage. Apply a sterile dressing or bandage to cover the wound. This protects it from contamination and promotes healing. If a sterile dressing is unavailable, use a clean cloth or towel as a temporary measure.

If the bleeding is severe, doesn't stop, or the wound appears deep and requires professional attention, it's vital to seek immediate medical help. Medical professionals can assess the injury, provide appropriate treatment, and determine if further interventions like stitches are necessary. Bleeding should never be taken lightly, and prompt action is crucial. By following these steps, you can effectively manage bleeding incidents and ensure the best possible care for yourself or others.

Burns

Burns can be painful and potentially serious injuries that require proper care and attention. This section will provide you with essential information on how to manage and treat burns effectively. Just like many serious injuries, burns are correlated with time. The longer the burn goes untreated, the worse it will get.

Start by assessing the severity of the burn. Burns are categorized into three levels: first-degree, second-degree, and third-degree. First-degree burns are superficial and usually involve redness and mild pain. Second-degree burns are deeper and may cause blisters and more intense pain. Third-degree burns are the most severe, involving damage to all layers of the skin and potentially underlying tissues. Seek immediate medical attention for second and third-degree burns.

For first-degree burns, cool the affected area under cool (not cold) running water for 10-20 minutes. This helps to reduce pain, prevent further damage, and promote healing. Avoid using ice or very cold water, as it can cause more harm. As a burn is open skin, make sure to use the cleanest water possible, as this will be an open source for bacteria and infection.

After cooling the burn, cover it with a sterile, non-stick dressing or clean cloth to protect it from infection. Avoid using adhesive bandages directly on the burn, as they can stick to the wound and cause further damage. If a sterile dressing is unavailable, a clean cloth or towel can be used temporarily.

Burns are excruciating and not always easy to relieve. Over-the-counter pain relievers, such as acetaminophen or ibuprofen, can help alleviate pain and reduce burn-related inflammation. Follow the recommended dosage instructions and consult a healthcare professional if needed, especially for burns involving children or severe pain.

As mentioned earlier, second-and third-degree burns require immediate medical attention. Additionally, seek medical help if the burn is larger than a small patch, shows signs of infection (redness, swelling, pus), or if you experience symptoms such as fever, increased pain, or worsening of the burn.

Burns should be handled with care and proper treatment to minimize complications and promote healing. By following these steps, you can effectively manage burns until professional medical help is available. Remember, seeking medical assistance is crucial for severe burns or burns that show signs of infection or worsening symptoms.

Fractures and Sprains

Unfortunately, in this section, there isn't much you can do for a fracture or sprain. However, everyone should know some simple and crucial things when it comes to the initial assessment of a possible fracture sprain.

Fractures and sprains are common injuries that can cause pain and limit mobility. This section will provide you with essential information on how to manage and treat fractures and sprains effectively.

Differentiating fractures and sprains:

Understanding the difference between fractures and sprains is crucial for proper management. A fracture refers to a broken bone, while a sprain refers to damage to ligaments surrounding a joint. Fractures often result from trauma, while sprains typically occur due to twisting or stretching of ligaments. Fractures involve a break or crack in a bone, resulting in pain, swelling, and deformity, with the potential for bone fragments to protrude. In contrast, sprains damage ligaments connecting bones, leading to swelling, bruising, and limited joint movement.

A key distinction lies in the nature of the injury; fractures exhibit localized pain at the site of the break, while sprains typically involve pain around the affected joint. Additionally, fractures may produce a grating or snapping sound upon injury, while sprains are often associated with a tearing sensation. Proper evaluation and understanding of these differences guide the application of first aid measures, which we will discuss in this next section.

Initial care:

For both fractures and sprains, it's essential to follow the RICE method:

- Rest: Avoid putting weight or strain on the injured area.
- Ice: Apply an ice pack or cold compress to reduce swelling and pain. Use it for about 15-20 minutes every few hours while ensuring a barrier (e.g., towel) between the ice and skin to prevent ice burns.
- Compression: Use an elastic bandage to wrap the injured area snugly but not too tight to help reduce swelling.
- Elevation: Keep the injured area elevated above heart level, if possible, to reduce swelling.

Seeking medical attention:

While minor sprains can often be managed at home, seeking medical attention for suspected fractures or severe sprains is essential. Signs that necessitate medical help include inability to bear weight or use the injured area, visible deformities, severe pain, or numbness and tingling.

Additionally, it's critical to get medical attention right away if there is chronic swelling and bruises, or if the injured joint seems misplaced. Getting medical help guarantees a complete assessment, precise diagnosis, and suitable therapy. Additionally, when fractures are suspected, medical practitioners can use imaging techniques like MRIs or X-rays to determine the degree of the damage. Prompt action on the part of medical professionals can aid in avoiding possible side effects like persistent discomfort, instability, or long-term joint damage. When first aid treatments are ineffective in reducing symptoms within a fair amount of time, it is essential to see a doctor to discuss more advanced treatment options, such as physical therapy or, in some situations, surgery. Recall that prompt and appropriate medical evaluation is essential to sprains' full recovery and rehabilitation process and guarantees the best potential outcome for the patient.

***Safety note: If a fracture becomes open, meaning the broken bone has perforated the skin, this is a true medical emergency and will always require treatment from a medical professional. You may apply a clean bandage to the area to keep the open site clean, but do not use the RICE method in this case. Be prepared for a more extended emergency visit.

Immobilization:

Fractures often require immobilization to promote proper healing. This can be achieved through splinting or casting. If a splint is needed, gently support the injured area using soft padding and secure it in place with a bandage or tape. Avoid putting pressure directly on the injured site.

Pain management:

For the treatment of pain resulting from sprains and fractures, over-the-counter medications like acetaminophen or nonsteroidal anti-inflammatory medicines (NSAIDs) like ibuprofen may be helpful. It is important to adhere to the recommended dose guidelines and take into account any specific medical problems or contraindications. Make sure the individual with the injury stays well-hydrated because dehydration might make their discomfort worse.

Even though these actions might aid in reducing discomfort right after an accident, it is crucial to stress that seeking the advice of a healthcare provider for a complete evaluation is essential. If required, they can recommend more potent painkillers and more focused pain management techniques. In addition to making the patient feel more comfortable overall, effectively managing pain also helps the patient follow prescribed rest and rehabilitation schedules, facilitating a quicker and more efficient healing process.

Fractures and sprains can be challenging, but they can heal effectively with proper care and treatment. By following these steps, you can effectively manage fractures and sprains until professional medical help is available. Remember, seeking medical assistance is crucial for suspected fractures or severe sprains.

Choking

Choking incidents can occur suddenly and pose a grave threat to an individual's life. Recognizing the signs of choking is crucial for timely intervention. A person who is choking may exhibit a sudden inability to breathe, panic, and an urgent need to grasp at their throat. They might be unable to speak or cough effectively, and the skin around their lips and fingertips may take on a bluish hue, signaling a lack of oxygen. In such cases, immediate action is essential.

If a person is speaking, talking, and vocalizing, this typically means the airway is still intact. As the individual may be uncomfortable and scared, this is a good sign the lodged object is not occluding the trachea. This can be even more true for children who have swallowed large pieces of unchewed food and have become lodged in the esophagus. Encourage the person to cough vigorously in these situations since it is a natural reaction that can assist in loosening the obstruction. If the victim is still breathing and able to speak, do not conduct any powerful abdominal thrusts or the Heimlich technique. Instead, be watchful, keep a constant eye on their condition, and be ready to take quick action if their speech becomes less frequent, if they cannot cough, or if their breathing becomes significantly impaired.

Even though a partial blockage is not as dangerous as a complete obstruction, it is still vital to seek expert assistance immediately. To make sure they get the proper care, call for emergency medical help. Maintaining composure, supporting the person, and exercising caution is critical since things can escalate quickly. The person's welfare should always come first, and you should always be prepared to act decisively when necessary.

Recognizing Choking:

When you identify someone choking, it's crucial to act swiftly. Encourage the person to cough forcefully to attempt to dislodge the obstructing object. If this proves ineffective, move on to the Heimlich maneuver. Be vigilant for signs of deterioration, such as loss of consciousness, and be prepared to initiate CPR if necessary. We will cover the CPR initiation process in a later step.

Always make sure to ask, "Are you choking?" As silly as it may sound, you do not want to be the person who performed a Heimlich maneuver on someone who isn't choking. People usually don't have kind words when the maneuver is misused.

Immediate Response:

The Heimlich maneuver is a primary response for choking in adults and children over one-year-old. To perform this maneuver, stand behind the person, place your arms around their waist, and form a fist with one hand. Position the fist just above the navel (that's the belly-button), grabbing it with your other hand, and deliver quick, upward thrusts. Continue these thrusts until the object is expelled or until emergency medical assistance arrives. If the person becomes unconscious, start CPR immediately, incorporating chest compressions and rescue breaths.

The Heimlich maneuver can be a highly effective technique, but it may need to be modified based on the individual's characteristics. For pregnant or obese individuals, place your hands higher on the chest, just below the breastbone, and perform firm, upward thrusts. Regular first aid training can help build the confidence to perform these maneuvers correctly in stressful situations, increasing the chances of a successful outcome. Remember, this is a quick and fast movement, not a crushing movement. The intention is for the person to expel the foreign object, not require emergency surgery from your Heimlich.

Choking in Infants:

Larger children may also receive the Heimlich as well, but choking incidents in infants necessitate a different approach. If an infant is choking, lay them face-down on your forearm, ensuring their head and neck are supported by your hand. Administer five firm back blows between the shoulder blades, followed by turning the infant over for chest compressions. It's vital to use a gentle but effective technique, considering the fragility of an infant's body. Many of their bones have not calcified the way our hardened adult bones have done in their maturing process.

Calling for Help and Continued Monitoring:

After successfully dislodging the obstructing object, or if emergency medical help is needed, call for professional assistance. Even if the individual appears to recover, it is crucial to seek medical attention to ensure there are no underlying issues or complications. Continue monitoring the individual for signs of shock, such as paleness, weakness, or altered consciousness, and provide reassurance until professional help arrives.

CHAPTER 4. CUTS, SCRAPES, AND WOUNDS:

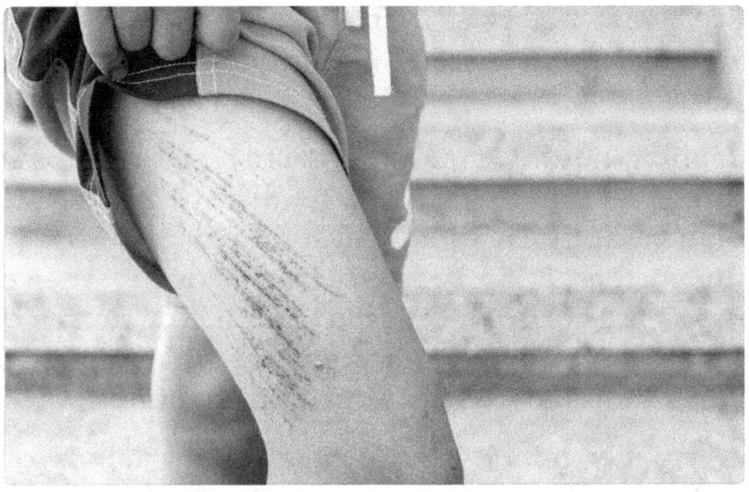

Life is inevitably messy, and even with the best intentions, accidents happen. Cuts, scrapes, and wounds, though often minor, are the body's way of sounding the alarm and alerting us to breaches in our protective barrier. Recognizing the different types of wounds and knowing how to handle them effectively is a crucial first aid skill, ensuring swift healing and minimizing the risk of complications.

It is also essential to understand the intricate process of blood clotting. It's a masterpiece of teamwork, orchestrated by your platelets and clotting factors, designed to seal leaks and prevent precious blood from spilling. Picture tiny platelets, the first responders rushing to the scene, sticking to the wound's edges, and forming a sticky plug. This initial dam slows the flow, buying time for reinforcements. Next, clotting factors, like proteins and enzymes, arrive on the scene, weaving a web of fibrin around the platelets, strengthening the barrier. Imagine this fibrin web as a delicate net, capturing more platelets and blood cells, building a sturdy clot that inhibits the flow.

But this clotting cascade is dynamic. It's like a construction crew that knows when to stop. Once the leak is plugged, enzymes dissolve the unnecessary fibrin, preventing the clot from growing into a problematic blockage. This balance between clotting and dissolving ensures efficient healing without compromising blood flow.

Understanding clotting empowers you to better care for wounds. Gentle pressure applied to the wound helps activate platelets and promotes clot formation. Elevation reduces blood pressure at the site, further minimizing bleeding. Knowing when clotting goes awry is crucial, too. Excessive bleeding or clotting beyond the wounded area might indicate more profound injuries or underlying conditions, requiring medical attention.

While seemingly minor, cuts, scrapes, and wounds can pose significant risks if not treated properly. Here's why they shouldn't be underestimated:

Infection: Open wounds are like welcome mats for bacteria, viruses, and other pathogens. If left untreated, these can cause infections, leading to redness, swelling, pain, and even severe complications like abscesses or sepsis. Infection can delay healing and potentially leave permanent scars.

Bleeding: Even small cuts can bleed significantly, leading to blood loss and dizziness, especially in children or individuals with underlying health conditions. Left unchecked, severe bleeding can be life-threatening.

Foreign objects: Cuts and scrapes can trap dirt, debris, or even glass or other sharp objects within the wound. These can cause further irritation, infection, and delay healing. Removing them can be painful and sometimes requires medical intervention.

Tetanus: Tetanus is a potentially fatal bacterial infection that enters the body through wounds. While vaccinations minimize the risk, neglecting proper wound care in at-risk individuals can lead to muscle spasms, breathing difficulties, and even death.

Underlying damage: Some seemingly minor cuts can conceal more profound damage to tendons, nerves, or blood vessels. Ignoring these can have long-term consequences, affecting movement, sensation, or even blood flow.

Remember, prompt and proper first aid for cuts, scrapes, and wounds can significantly reduce these risks, ensure faster healing, and prevent potential complications. This is why understanding wound cleaning, applying pressure to stop bleeding, and knowing when to seek medical attention are crucial first-aid skills to include in this book.

Assessing the Severity: From Minor Nicks to Deeper Cuts

Not all wounds are created equal. Some are mere paper cuts, leaving behind a thin red line that barely qualifies as a nuisance. Others, however, can be deep gashes, jagged tears, or even puncture wounds from sharp objects. Recognizing the severity of a wound is the first step in determining the appropriate course of action.

Minor wounds:

- Superficial cuts and scrapes less than ¼ inch deep
- Bleeding is minimal and easily controlled with direct pressure

Moderate wounds:

- Cuts deeper than ¼ inch, but less than ½ inch
- Bleeding may be moderate and require additional pressure or a pressure bandage
- It may have jagged edges or involve fatty tissue

Serious wounds:

- Deep cuts exceeding ½ inch or involving muscle, tendons, or nerves
- Heavy bleeding that doesn't respond to pressure
- Puncture wounds from sharp objects like nails or knives
- Open wounds exposing internal organs or bone

Remember: If you are unsure about the severity of a wound, always err on the side of caution and seek professional medical attention.

First Aid Essentials: Cleaning, Protecting, and Promoting Healing

Once the severity is assessed, it's time to take action. Proper wound care minimizes the risk of infection and promotes faster healing. Here's your first-aid toolkit in action:

Cleaning:

- **Wash your hands thoroughly** with soap and water to avoid transferring bacteria to the wound. Hand sanitizer is also a great alternative if you are unable to wash your hands properly. Sanitizers should always be 70% or greater in alcohol content to effectively sanitize your hands.
- **Flush the wound** gently with clean running water or sterile saline solution to remove dirt and debris. If using water, it should come from a clean source to minimize adding more contamination to the wound. Always go generously on the flushing side rather than the minimal side.
- **Pat the wound dry** with a clean, lint-free cloth or gauze

pad. Avoid rubbing and coated-gauze, as this can irritate the wound further.

Protecting the Wound

1. Pressure Points: Locate the pressure point nearest the wound and apply firm, steady pressure with a clean cloth or gauze pad directly over the bleeding source. Hold for several minutes, applying consistent pressure even if the bleeding seems to slow. If the cloth becomes soaked, apply another layer on top without removing the first. Remember, patience is key!

2. Elevation Advantage: Elevate the injured area above the heart whenever possible. This reduces blood flow to the wound, minimizing bleeding and promoting clotting. Use pillows, cushions, or even your own body to prop up the injured area comfortably.

3. Bandage Barricade: Once the bleeding slows, apply a breathable bandage to protect the wound from further contamination. Choose a size and material appropriate for the injury, ensuring it covers the wound edges without being too tight to restrict blood flow. Avoid using adhesive bandages directly on open wounds; opt for sterile gauze pads secured with non-adhesive tape or cloth ties. Remember, changing the bandage regularly is crucial for keeping the wound clean and promoting healing.

Promoting Healing:

1. Cleanliness is Key: Wash your hands thoroughly with soap and water before touching the wound or changing the bandage. Gently clean the wound with sterile saline solution or mild soap and water, avoiding harsh scrubbing. Pat dry with a clean, lint-free cloth.

2. Scabs: Resist the urge to pick at scabs! They are your body's natural protective barrier, shielding the wound from infection and promoting healing underneath. Picking at scabs can delay healing, increase the risk of scarring, and introduce bacteria into the wound.

3. Watchful Eye: Keep a close eye on the wound for signs of infection, including redness, swelling, pus drainage, or fever. These can be indicators of serious complications. If you notice any of these symptoms, don't hesitate to seek medical attention immediately. Early diagnosis and treatment of infection are crucial for optimal healing and preventing further health risks.

Remember, patience is a virtue when it comes to healing. While these steps offer a roadmap to recovery, every wound heals at its own pace. Listen to your body, prioritize rest, and follow any additional instructions a healthcare professional provides. You can guide your body towards a smooth and complete recovery with proper care and attention.

Other Measures:

Infections:

For minor cuts and scrapes, applying a thin layer of antibiotic ointment can help prevent bacterial infections. Choose one with ingredients like bacitracin or polymyxin B, avoiding products with unnecessary fragrances or dyes. Remember, antibiotics won't heal the wound. They help prevent infections from taking hold.

Pain:

Over-the-counter pain relievers like ibuprofen or acetaminophen can effectively manage discomfort associated with minor injuries. Follow dosage instructions carefully and consult a healthcare professional if the pain is severe or persistent. Remember, pain is a signal from your body, so pay attention to its intensity and seek medical advice if needed.

Tetanus:

Get your tetanus shots up to date! Tetanus is a rare but potentially fatal bacterial infection that enters the body through wounds. Ensure your tetanus vaccination is current, typically recommended every 10 years, to shield yourself from this preventable threat.

Cuts, Scrapes, and Beyond: Recognizing Other Types of Wounds

While cuts and scrapes are common, other types of wounds require specific attention:

- **Puncture wounds:** Deep, narrow wounds caused by sharp objects like nails or knives. These wounds can be particularly prone to infection due to the difficulty of cleaning them thoroughly. Seek medical attention for all puncture wounds.
- **Burns:** Thermal injuries caused by heat, chemicals, or electricity. The severity of a burn depends on the depth and extent of the injury. Apply cool compresses to minor burns and seek immediate medical attention for severe burns.
- **Animal bites:** Bites from animals can carry a high risk of infection and rabies. Clean the wound thoroughly and seek medical attention immediately.

Remember, Knowledge is Power: When in Doubt, Seek Help

While this chapter provides a basic framework for managing cuts, scrapes, and other minor wounds, remember that first aid is a complex skill best learned through proper training and certification. When faced with a serious wound or any uncertainties, always err on the side of caution and seek professional medical attention. Your health and well-being are worth it.

CHAPTER 5: BURNS AND SCALDS

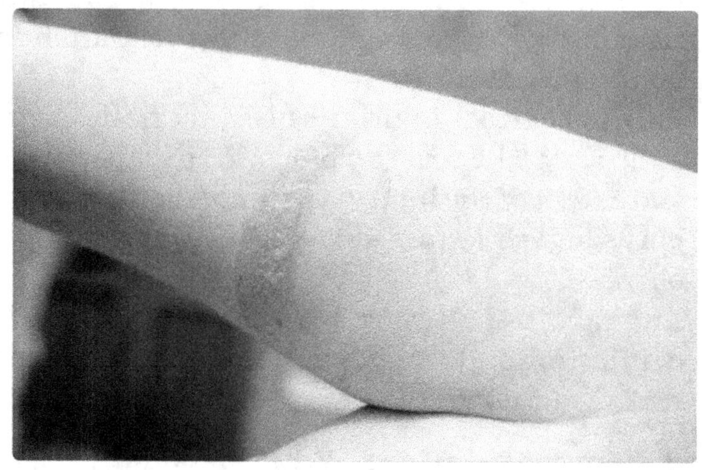

Burns and scalds caused by exposure to heat, chemicals, or electricity are no laughing matter. They can range from mild discomfort to life-threatening injuries, demanding swift and appropriate action. This chapter equips you with the knowledge to navigate the flames, providing crucial information on treating burns, managing pain, and recognizing when to seek medical assistance.

Understanding the Burn Spectrum: From Sunburns to Serious Injuries

The first step in managing a burn is understanding its severity. Burns are classified based on the depth of tissue damage:

- **First-degree burns:** Affect the outermost layer of skin (epidermis), causing redness, pain, and swelling. Sunburns are a typical example.

- **Second-degree burns:** Damage the epidermis and part of the dermis (second layer of skin), resulting in blistering, redness, and severe pain.

- **Third-degree burns:** Destroy the entire epidermis and dermis, often charring or leathery in appearance. These burns are painless due to nerve damage but require immediate medical attention.

- **Fourth-degree burns:** Extend through all skin layers, damaging underlying tissues like muscle and bone. These are life-threatening injuries and require immediate medical intervention.

Immediate Response: The Golden Minutes of Burn Care

The first few minutes after a burn are crucial. Quick action minimizes tissue damage and promotes healing. Here's what to do:

1. Stop the Burning Process:

- **Fire:** Act decisively to remove the source of heat. Smother flames with a thick cloth, throw water or sand, or utilize fire extinguishers if available. Don't attempt to use yourself as a shield; protect yourself first.
- **Chemicals:** Flush the area with clean, running water for at least 20 minutes to remove any lingering chemicals that might continue to burn the skin. Wear gloves if available to protect yourself from contamination.

2. Cool the Burn:

- Cool, Not Cold: Immerse the burn in cool (not ice-cold)

water for at least 20 minutes. Cooler water can soothe the pain and stop the burning process from progressing further. Avoid using ice directly on the burn, as it can worsen tissue damage.

- Gentle Flow: If submerging isn't practical, apply cool compresses soaked in water or saline solution. Change the compresses frequently to maintain consistent cooling. Remember, continuous cooling is critical in the first few hours after a burn.

3. Free the Bound:

- Clothing Conundrum: Gently remove any clothing or jewelry that might trap heat or constrict the burned area. If clothing sticks to the skin, don't attempt to tear it off, as this can cause further damage. If possible, cut around the burned area and leave the stuck parts alone until professional medical attention is available.
- Bling Beware: Remove rings, bracelets, or necklaces, especially if swelling is already occurring. Tight, constricting jewelry can impede blood flow to the burned area and worsen the injury.

Soothe the Burn:

- Apply a loose, sterile dressing or clean cloth to the burn. Avoid tight bandages that can restrict blood flow.
- Elevate the burned area above the heart if possible to reduce swelling.

Manage Pain:

- Over-the-counter pain relievers like ibuprofen or acetaminophen can help manage discomfort.

Seek Medical Attention When Needed:

While minor first-degree burns can be treated at home, seek immediate medical attention for:

- Second-degree burns larger than your hand
- Third-degree burns (any size)
- Chemical or electrical burns
- Burns on the face, hands, feet, genitals, or joints
- Burns in infants or elderly individuals
- Any burn causing difficulty breathing, severe pain, or signs of infection

Bonus Tips for Burn Care:

- Don't break blisters: Blisters protect the wound from infection. Let them drain naturally.
- Avoid applying ointments or creams unless instructed by a doctor.
- Stay hydrated: Burns can lead to dehydration. Drink plenty of fluids.
- Prevent infection: Keep the burn clean and covered with a bandage until healed.

Remember: Burns are serious injuries. When in doubt, always seek medical attention.

House Fires

Even though this may stray a little from the burns chapter, it brings many important concepts to discuss since a house fire can happen to any of us when we least expect it. Many products generate heat and extreme temperatures in our homes, and we can have a combustible situation with the perfect conditions (heat, oxygen, and a fuel source). While immediate burn treatment is crucial, the first priority in any house fire should always be escape and ensuring everyone's safety. Here's what to remember if you find yourself facing this harrowing situation:

Act Fast, Think Clear:

- Don't waste time: Every second counts when escaping a fire. Stay calm, follow established fire escape plans, and evacuate immediately using designated emergency exits. If you haven't designated an escape route with yourself or family members, now is the time to have something in writing.

Know Your Exits:

- Familiarity is key: Have a pre-planned escape route in place and ensure everyone in your household is familiar with it. Practice drills regularly to act on instinct in an emergency.

Stay Low, Go Slow:

- Smoke and heat rise: As a fire blazes, this can build exceptionally quickly in a home, making it almost unbearable to push forward. Crawl on your hands and knees below the smoke to avoid choking fumes and navigate towards your escape route.

Close Doors Behind You:

- Contain the flames: Closing doors can slow the spread of fire and allow others more time to escape. Do not lock doors behind you while others are still inside.

If Trapped:

- Seek refuge: If escape is impossible, find a safe, enclosed room with a door you can close and stuff with towels or blankets to block smoke. Call emergency services immediately and wait for rescue.

Inhalation Burns: The Hidden Danger:

- Invisible Threat: Even in minor fires, smoke inhalation can cause serious, often invisible, lung damage. Be aware of coughing, difficulty breathing, or dizziness, which can indicate smoke inhalation even if burns are not apparent.
- **Airway Burns**: With high heat, the airways are susceptible to this and can cause the same swelling and

irritation as our skin. In case of airway swelling, it is essential to seek medical attention after a house fire.

Seek Medical Attention:

Don't ignore the unseen: After escaping a fire, seek immediate medical attention to assess for potential inhalation injuries, even if you feel well. Early diagnosis and treatment can prevent complications. Whether it is smoke inhalation, burns, or toxic fumes, you will want to be checked out by a medical professional.

Living Beyond the Burn: Scarring and Emotional Trauma

Burns can leave physical and emotional scars. While some scarring is inevitable, proper wound care and treatments like silicone gel sheets can minimize their appearance. Additionally, don't underestimate the emotional impact of burns. Seek support from therapists or burn survivor groups to navigate the healing process holistically.

By understanding burns, acting swiftly, and seeking appropriate medical help, you can significantly improve the outcome of these fiery encounters. Remember, knowledge is power – arm yourself with it and face burns with confidence and care.

CHAPTER 6: FRACTURES, SPRAINS, AND STRAINS

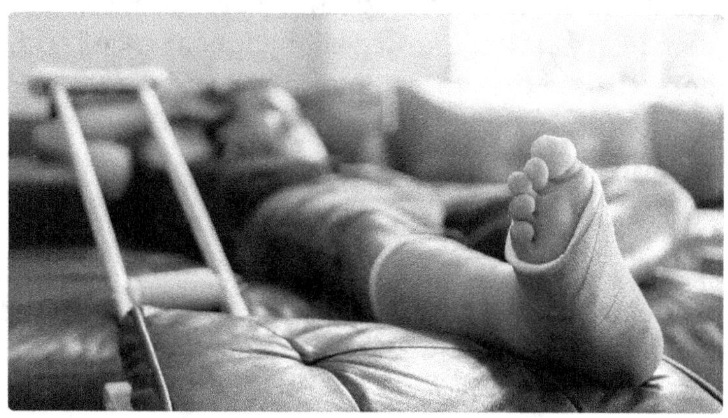

Whether it's a misstep on the uneven sidewalk or an enthusiastic sports play gone wrong, bone and muscle injuries can send shivers down anyone's spine. But fear not! This chapter equips you with the knowledge to distinguish between fractures, sprains, and strains, administer vital first aid, and determine when professional help is needed.

The Bony Puzzle: Recognizing Fractures

Fractures, or broken bones, come in various forms, each requiring specific attention. Here's how to identify the telltale signs:

- **Bone deformity:** The affected limb might appear visibly bent, twisted, or shortened.

- **Severe pain:** Fractures often cause intense, localized pain that worsens with movement.
- **Swelling and bruising:** Fractured areas typically experience significant swelling and discoloration around the injury site.
- **Loss of function:** Fractures often make it difficult or impossible to move the affected limb normally.
- **Grating sensation:** In some cases, you might feel or hear a grating sensation when moving the broken bone.

Remember: Not all fractures are obvious. If you suspect a bone break, even without immediate visible signs, seek medical attention promptly. Early diagnosis and treatment are crucial for optimal healing and minimizing complications.

Sprains and Strains: When Ligaments and Muscles Cry Out

While fractures involve bone, sprains and strains target the soft tissues that support and connect them. Here's how to tell them apart:

- **Sprains:** These involve stretched or torn ligaments, the tough bands connecting bones at joints. Sprains typically occur around ankles, knees, and wrists.

- **Strains:** These involve overstretched or torn muscles or tendons (muscle-to-bone connectors). Back, hamstring, and shoulder strains are common.

Common signs of both sprains and strains include:

- **Pain:** Localized pain that worsens with movement.
- **Swelling and tenderness:** The affected area becomes puffy and feels sensitive to touch.
- **Bruising:** Discoloration may appear around the injury site.
- **Reduced mobility:** Moving the affected limb becomes difficult or painful.

The RICE Formula: Your First Aid Weapon

While fractures call for immediate medical attention, sprains and strains can often be managed with the RICE protocol:

- **Rest:** Immobilize the injured area to prevent further damage. Use splints, slings, or crutches as needed.
- **Ice:** Apply ice packs wrapped in a towel to the affected area for 15-20 minutes at a time, several times a day, to reduce swelling and pain.
- **Compression:** Use an elastic bandage (not too tight!) to provide support and minimize swelling.
- **Elevation:** Keep the injured limb elevated above the heart to reduce swelling and promote drainage.

Seeking Help: When RICE Isn't Enough

While RICE is effective for many sprains and strains, some situations demand professional intervention:

- Severe pain that doesn't improve with RICE
- Significant swelling or deformity
- Inability to bear weight on the injured limb
- Numbness or tingling in the affected area
- Open wounds or visible bone fragments (indicating a possible fracture)

Bonus Tips:

- **Stay hydrated:** Proper hydration promotes healing and reduces inflammation.
- **Maintain a healthy diet:** Nourish your body with essential nutrients for optimal repair.
- **Follow doctor's instructions:** If necessary, adhere to prescribed medications or physical therapy for faster recovery.

Remember, fractures, sprains, and strains require different approaches. While RICE can be your first-line defense for sprains and strains, **fractures demand immediate medical attention.** By understanding the signs, administering appropriate first aid, and seeking professional help, you can confidently navigate these musculoskeletal mishaps and pave the way for a speedy recovery.

CHAPTER 7: ALLERGIC REACTIONS AND ANAPHYLAXIS

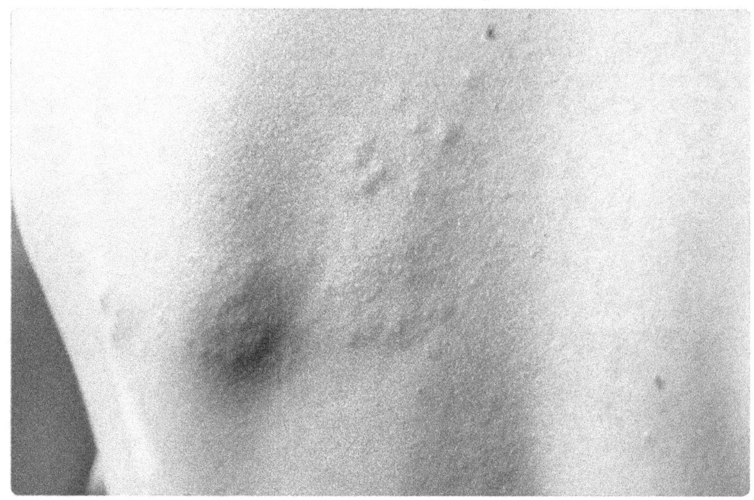

From pollen's playful sneezes to shellfish's life-threatening sting, allergies are the immune system's misguided attempts at protecting us from perceived threats. This chapter equips you with the knowledge to navigate the terrain of allergies, recognize their symptoms, administer relief measures, and identify when to seek immediate medical attention for severe reactions like anaphylaxis.

Our bodies can react to an extensive array of seemingly harmless and downright scary substances. Common allergens include:

- **Food:** Peanuts, shellfish, eggs, dairy, soy, and tree nuts top the list.

- **Inhalants:** Pollen, dust mites, mold, and pet dander are frequent culprits in seasonal and year-round allergies.

- **Insect stings:** Bee stings, wasp stings, and mosquito bites can trigger allergic reactions in some individuals.

- **Medications:** Antibiotics, aspirin, and certain pain relievers can trigger allergic reactions.

Allergic Reactions:

Imagine a bustling city bustling with activity, constantly on guard against invaders. That's your immune system, a microscopic metropolis working tirelessly to keep you healthy. From sniffles to scrapes, it's the silent hero defending your body against viruses, bacteria, and other unwelcome guests. Here's a glimpse into its fascinating workings:

The Two-Pronged Defense:

Your immune system operates on two levels: the innate immune system and the adaptive immune system. Think of the innate system as the city walls, providing a rapid, non-specific defense against intruders. It includes:

- Physical barriers: Skin, mucus membranes, and even tears act as the initial guard, preventing germs from entering your body.
- Phagocytes: These warrior cells gobble up invading bacteria and viruses, breaking them down for disposal.
- Inflammation: Redness, swelling, and warmth are signs of the immune system rallying its troops to fight infection.

The adaptive immune system, on the other hand, is like a special forces unit, meticulously recognizing and targeting specific threats. It forms "memory cells" after each encounter, building up a customized arsenal to fight off future invasions of the same enemy.

The Battle Plan:

When a germ breaks through the initial defenses, the adaptive system swings into action:

- Antigen Recognition: Special white blood cells called B cells and T cells identify unique "flags" (antigens) on the germs, distinguishing them from healthy cells.
- Antibody Production: B cells churn out proteins called antibodies, each uniquely shaped to latch onto a specific antigen, like a lock and key.
- Neutralization: Once locked on, antibodies neutralize the germs, marking them for destruction by phagocytes or rendering them harmless.
- Memory Formation: Some B and T cells become memory cells, remembering the specific antigen and gearing up for a faster response if the same germ attacks again.

Keeping the Peace:

Once the foreign object to the body is removed, the immune system winds down, but it never sleeps. It constantly patrols your body, scanning for potential threats and keeping you healthy.

When the immune system encounters an allergen, it mistakenly identifies it as a harmful invader. This triggers the release of histamine and other chemicals, leading to a cascade of unpleasant symptoms:

- **Mild reactions:** Runny nose, sneezing, itchy eyes, skin rashes, mild nausea, and stomach cramps are common occurrences.

- **Moderate reactions:** Difficulty breathing, wheezing, vomiting, diarrhea, and swelling of the lips, tongue, or throat can indicate a more severe reaction.

- **Anaphylaxis:** A life-threatening reaction leading to the rapid onset of severe symptoms like airway closure, shock, and even cardiac arrest. Requires immediate medical attention!

Antihistamines: The First Line of Defense

Over-the-counter antihistamines like Allegra, Zyrtec, and Benadryl can be your first line of defense against mild to moderate allergic reactions. These medications block the action of histamine, alleviating symptoms like sneezing, itching, and hives.

Remember: Antihistamines are not a substitute for seeking medical attention in case of severe allergic reactions or anaphylaxis.

The EpiPen: A Lifesaving Ally in Anaphylaxis

For individuals with a history of severe allergic reactions or anaphylaxis, carrying an EpiPen is crucial. This auto-injector delivers a predetermined dose of epinephrine, a hormone that rapidly counteracts the effects of an allergic reaction, opening airways and restoring blood pressure.

Using an EpiPen:

1. **Recognize the signs of anaphylaxis:** Difficulty breathing, wheezing, swelling, dizziness, and rapid heartbeat are red flags.
2. **Remove the allergen if possible.**
3. **Call emergency services immediately.**
4. **Administer the EpiPen injection according to manufacturer instructions.** Hold the device firmly against the thigh and press the injector firmly.
5. **Lay the person flat on their back with legs elevated.**

6. **Monitor the person's condition until medical help arrives.**

Remember: Even after administering an EpiPen, stay with the person and continue monitoring their condition until medical professionals arrive.

Living with Allergies: Knowledge is Power

By understanding common allergens, recognizing symptoms, and knowing how to respond to mild and severe reactions, you can navigate the world of allergies with confidence.

Remember:

- **Early identification and avoidance of triggers are crucial to preventing allergic reactions.**
- **Always carry an EpiPen and know how to use it if you are at risk for anaphylaxis.**
- **Consult with a healthcare professional for proper diagnosis, treatment plans, and allergy management strategies.**

With the proper knowledge and tools, allergies don't have to hold you back. Embrace life's adventures, armed with awareness and prepared to combat any unwelcome immune system surprises.

I hope this chapter empowers you to navigate the world of allergies with confidence and knowledge. Feel free to ask any further questions you may have about specific allergens, symptom management, or emergency protocols for anaphylaxis. Remember, knowledge is power – use it to be your own allergy-fighting champion!

CHAPTER 8: CHOKING AND CPR

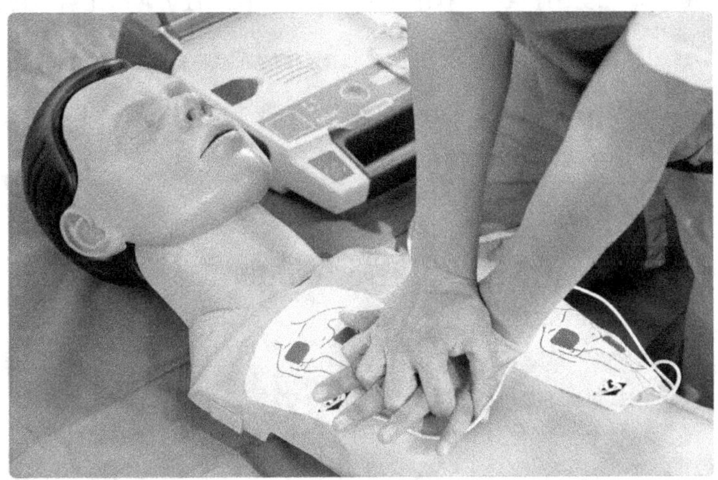

Life is full of unexpected moments, and knowing how to react in one where another's life hangs in the balance can be the difference between tragedy and triumph. This chapter equips you with the knowledge to act swiftly and effectively in two critical situations: choking and cardiac arrest. By mastering the Heimlich maneuver and CPR, you become a potential lifesaver, ready to spring into action and deliver the breath of life when needed.

Choking: Recognizing the Silent Struggle

Choking occurs when an object blocks the airway, preventing oxygen from reaching the lungs. Early recognition and intervention are crucial. Watch for these telltale signs:

- **Inability to speak or breathe:** Choking victims often grasp their throat or clutch at their chest, unable to form words or make sounds.
- **Universal choking sign:** A person will naturally grab towards their neck and become physically distraught when something becomes lodged in the throat. Holding both hands above the head with thumbs and index fingers forming a circle is a universal signal for choking.
- **Facial expressions:** Panic, distress, and grimacing facial expressions can further indicate airway obstruction.

The Heimlich Maneuver: Your Choking Countermeasure

If someone is choking, act quickly and decisively. Here's how to perform the Heimlich maneuver:

For adults and children above one-year-old:

1. Stand behind the person and wrap your arms around their waist.
2. Place a fist with one hand just below the sternum (breastbone), between the rib cage and belly button.
3. Grasp your fist with your other hand and deliver a quick, upward thrust to expel the object from the airway.
4. Repeat thrusts until the object dislodges or the person starts breathing and coughing.

For infants (less than one-year-old):

1. Lay the infant face down on your forearm, supporting their head and neck with your hand.
2. Deliver five sharp back blows between the shoulder blades using the heel of your other hand.
3. Turn the infant face up and place two fingers in the center of their breastbone.
4. Deliver five chest compressions, pushing straight down about 1.5 inches.
5. Repeat the cycle of back blows and chest compressions

until the object dislodges or the infant starts breathing.

Remember: If the Heimlich maneuver fails after several attempts, call emergency services immediately and continue trying until help arrives. If you do not feel a pulse and the person is unconscious, begin CPR!

CPR: Pumping Life Back into a Still Heart

Cardiac arrest occurs when the heart stops beating effectively, cutting off blood flow to vital organs. CPR helps by artificially pumping blood and providing oxygen to the brain and other organs until medical help arrives.

Performing CPR:

1. **Check for responsiveness:** Tap the person and ask loudly if they are okay. If they don't respond, call emergency services and start CPR immediately. Make sure you have called or designated someone to call 911 at this point. It is usually better to designate so you can begin CPR as soon as possible.
2. **Place the person on a firm surface.**
3. **Kneel beside them and locate the center of their chest, between the nipples.**
4. **Feel for a pulse:** Feel for a pulse firmly, but not aggressively, under the chin and to either side of the neck. This should be done for 5 seconds, but no longer than 10 seconds.
5. **Place the heel of your dominant hand on the center of the chest, and place your other hand on top, interlacing your fingers.**
6. **Position your shoulders directly over your hands and keep your elbows straight.**
7. **Push down hard and fast, compressing the chest at least 2 inches (5 centimeters) but no more than 2.4 inches (6 centimeters).**
8. **Aim for a rate of 100 to 120 compressions per minute.**

> **You can use the song "Stayin' Alive" to maintain the correct rhythm.**

9. **After every 30 chest compressions, deliver two rescue breaths** (*as getting oxygen into the body is crucial to sustaining life; if you are uncomfortable with providing rescue breaths, continue with chest compressions until emergency services arrive*).

10. **Tilt the head back slightly and pinch the soft part of the nose closed.**

11. **Seal your mouth over the person's mouth and give two breaths, each lasting about one second, watching for the chest to rise with each breath.**

12. **Continue cycles of 30 chest compressions followed by two rescue breaths until the person starts breathing on their own, help arrives, or you are too exhausted to continue.**

Introducing the AED

CPR is a vital tool in every first-aider's arsenal, but sometimes, even the most dedicated chest compressions and rescue breaths need a helping hand. This is where the AED, or Automated External Defibrillator, steps in. Think of it as a portable electrical jolt capable of restarting a chaotic heart rhythm back into a life-saving beat.

Bonus Tip: There are only two shockable rhythms: Ventricular tachycardia (V-Tach and ventricular fibrillation (V-Fib). You are not expected to know these, which is beyond this book's scope, but understand that not all cardiac arrests are shockable, so the AED may not shock if it doesn't detect these rhythms.

When to Call on the AED:

- Sudden Cardiac Arrest: The key word here is "sudden." If someone collapses unexpectedly and isn't breathing normally, cardiac arrest is a strong possibility.
- Unresponsive and Not Breathing: Check for

responsiveness and breathing for no more than 10 seconds. If there's no response and no normal breathing, start CPR immediately.

- AED Available: If an AED is readily available, retrieve it while someone continues CPR. Don't delay CPR to fetch the AED unless it's immediately nearby.

AED in Action:

- Clear the Area: Ensure no one is touching the victim and call for emergency services if not already done.
- Follow the Prompts: The AED is designed for ease of use, with clear instructions and voice commands guiding you through the process. Apply the electrode pads as directed, typically one on the chest and one on the back.
- Analyze and Advise: The AED will analyze the victim's heart rhythm and determine if a shock is necessary. It will clearly tell you if a shock is advised and guide you through delivering it if needed.
- Continue CPR: After each shock, or if no shock is advised, continue CPR for 2 minutes before the AED reanalyzes the rhythm. Repeat this cycle until emergency personnel arrive.

Key Points:

- Don't be intimidated: AEDs are designed for anyone to use, regardless of medical training. Trust the clear instructions and remain calm.
- Don't delay: Early defibrillation significantly increases the chances of survival. Don't hesitate to use the AED if available.
- CPR remains crucial: Even with an AED, consistent CPR provides vital blood flow to the brain and organs until a normal rhythm is restored.

The AED is a powerful tool in the fight against sudden cardiac arrest, but it's not a magic bullet. It works best alongside your quick action and commitment to effective CPR. By equipping yourself with both skills and the knowledge of AED use, you can become a true lifesaver, ready to step in when a heart needs a second chance.

When Not to Perform CPR: Prioritizing Safety and Respect

CPR is a lifesaving procedure, but it's important to understand that it's not always necessary or appropriate. Performing CPR in certain situations can be harmful and even violate the individual's wishes. Here are some key scenarios where CPR should *not* be initiated:

- Obvious Signs of Death: If the person displays clear signs of rigor mortis (stiffening of the body), decomposition, or profound head trauma, CPR will not be effective. Respect their final state and focus on comfort measures for loved ones present.

- Obvious Signs of Life: I know this may seem like a no-brainer, but if a person is awake and speaking (versus unconscious and non-responsive), do not start CPR on this person. You could unintentionally put someone into an actual cardiac arrest.

- Confirmed Death by Medical Professionals: If a doctor or other qualified medical personnel has declared the deceased, do not attempt CPR. Their training and experience equip them to make this determination accurately.

- Terminal Illness with Palliative Care: If the person is in the final stages of a terminal illness and receiving appropriate palliative care, their wishes may involve a peaceful passing without aggressive interventions like CPR. Honor their choices and focus on offering emotional support.

- Unsafe Scene: If the scene is unsafe for you or others due to fire, electrical hazards, or ongoing violence, do not attempt CPR. Prioritize your own safety and that of others before attempting any medical interventions.

- Advanced Directives: Some individuals may have expressed their wishes through documents like living wills or Do Not Resuscitate (DNR) orders. These documents legally instruct medical professionals not to perform CPR in the event of cardiac arrest. Respect their wishes and avoid unnecessary interventions.

Remember: Always prioritize your own safety and the safety of others. If you are trying to decide whether or not to perform CPR, err on the side of caution and seek help from qualified medical professionals. Their expertise and judgment will guide you toward the most appropriate course of action.

Remember:

- Early CPR can significantly increase the chances of survival from cardiac arrest.
- Do not hesitate to start CPR even if you haven't been formally trained, but I always suggest getting trained, as it is a valuable skill that will last a lifetime.
- Modifications may be needed for CPR on infants and children. Consult trained professionals for specific instructions.
- Always initiate an emergency response (dial 911 in America) by you or a fellow witness so help is on the way.
- If an AED is available, make sure to utilize it. It will prompt you on what to do.

Knowledge is Power, Action is Life-Saving

Knowing how to handle choking and perform CPR empowers you to act as a first responder in critical situations. This knowledge can literally be the difference between life and death for someone in your path. Remember, practice makes perfect. Consider enrolling in CPR and first aid training courses to refine your skills and ensure confidence in your ability to act when needed.

CHAPTER 9: POISONING AND OVERDOSES

The home, meant to be a haven, can unexpectedly harbor hidden dangers in the form of household chemicals and medications. Accidental ingestions and overdoses can occur in the blink of an eye, leaving loved ones scrambling for solutions. This chapter equips you with the knowledge to identify common household poisons, manage accidental ingestions, and provide initial care for drug overdoses, empowering you to navigate the toxic maze and be prepared for the unthinkable. *Understand that most poisonings and overdoses will require emergency services, as many will require higher levels of medical care.* However, there are steps we can all take to minimize the injuries from one.

Unmasking the Toxic Villains: Common Household Poisons

Everyday household items, from seemingly harmless cleaning products to medications within reach, can pose serious threats if ingested. Some of the most common culprits include:

- **Cleaning products:** Bleach, drain cleaners, oven cleaners, disinfectants, and laundry detergents can cause burns, respiratory distress, and organ damage.

- **Pain relievers:** Over-the-counter pain medications like ibuprofen and acetaminophen, when ingested in excess, can lead to liver damage, kidney failure, and respiratory problems.

- **Prescription medications:** Antidepressants, sedatives, and blood thinners can cause serious side effects and even death if taken in unintended amounts.

- **Plants:** Many common houseplants like lilies, poinsettias, and dieffenbachia can be toxic if ingested, causing vomiting, diarrhea, and even seizures.

- **Chemicals:** Pesticides, antifreeze, and gasoline are highly toxic and can cause severe organ damage or death if ingested, even in small amounts.

Signs of Trouble: Recognizing Symptoms of Ingestion

Early identification of poisoning is crucial. Be alert for these warning signs:

- **Nausea and vomiting**
- **Diarrhea**

- **Abdominal pain**
- **Dizziness and confusion**
- **Difficulty breathing**
- **Seizures**
- **Loss of consciousness**

First Steps in Poisoning: Acting Swiftly and Safely

If you suspect an accidental ingestion, stay calm and act quickly. Here's what to do:

1. Identify the poison: If possible, determine the substance ingested and the amount consumed.
2. Call emergency services immediately.
3. Do not induce vomiting unless instructed by a medical professional.
4. If the poison is on the skin or clothing, remove contaminated clothing and flush the area with clean water for at least 15 minutes.
5. Stay with the person and monitor their condition until help arrives.

Important Note: Never try to diagnose or treat poisoning yourself. Always seek immediate medical attention.

Overdoses: When Medications Become Monsters

Drug overdoses can occur accidentally or intentionally, leading to life-threatening situations. Be aware of these warning signs:

- **Drowsiness and confusion**
- **Shallow or slow breathing**
- **Blue-tinged skin or lips**
- **Loss of consciousness**
- **Seizures**
- **Vomiting with blood**

Responding to an Overdose: Time is of the Essence

If you suspect a drug overdose, act swiftly and decisively:

1. **Call emergency services immediately.**
2. **If the person is unconscious, check for breathing and pulse.**
3. **If they are not breathing, start CPR.**
4. **Do not try to induce vomiting.**
5. **Stay with the person and monitor their condition until help arrives.**

Prevention is Key: Minimizing the Risk

The best way to deal with poisoning and overdoses is to prevent them in the first place. Here are some essential tips:

- Store all medications and household chemicals safely, out of reach of children and pets.
- Keep medication bottles in their original containers. This includes child-safety lids properly in place.
- Do not share medications with others.
- Do not take medication without knowing what it is (missing labels, damaged labels, mixed medication, etc.)
- Dispose of unused medications properly.
- Teach children about the dangers of ingesting unknown substances.
- Install childproof locks on cabinets and drawers where dangerous items are stored.

By being aware of common houshold poisons, recognizing symptoms of ingestions and overdoses, and taking preventive measures, you can significantly reduce the risk of poisoning and equip yourself to handle an emergency with confidence and clarity. Remember, your knowledge and swift action can make all the difference when it comes to protecting yourself and your loved ones from the unforeseen dangers lurking within the seemingly familiar walls of your home.

CHAPTER 10: EMERGENCY PREPAREDNESS

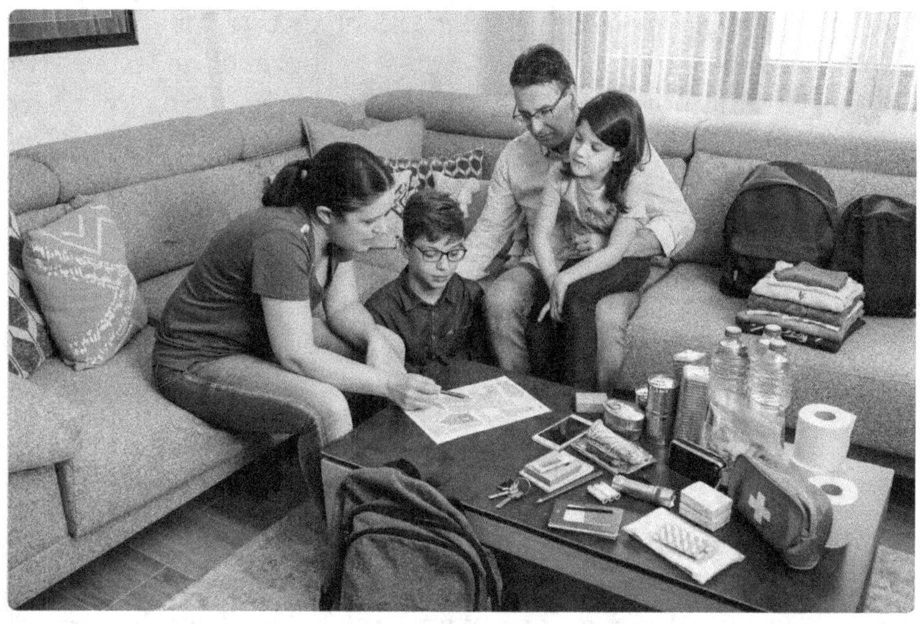

The world is a dynamic place, with nature's unpredictability occasionally throwing curveballs that disrupt our routine. From raging floods to crippling blizzards, natural disasters can test our resilience and push us to our limits. However, within this uncertainty lies the power of preparedness. This chapter equips you with the knowledge and practical tips to transform your home into a haven of resilience in any emergency.

Building a Fortress of Foresight: Crafting an Emergency Plan

Before the storm clouds gather, take proactive steps by creating a comprehensive emergency plan. This blueprint for action ensures everyone knows what to do when disaster strikes:

- **Identify potential threats:** Assess your location's vulnerability to natural disasters like floods, earthquakes, storms, or power outages.
- **Designate escape routes:** Determine multiple evacuation routes out of your home and neighborhood, accounting for potential road closures or blockages.
- **Choose meeting points:** Establish two meeting points – one outside your home for immediate evacuation and another outside your neighborhood for long-term regrouping.
- **Assign roles and responsibilities:** Delegate tasks like communication, emergency kit maintenance, and first aid amongst family members. This can include older siblings being in charge of directing younger siblings to designated areas. Having a neighbor you feel comfortable for your family to be directed to is also an excellent way for everyone to escape danger and have a meeting spot in an emergency.
- **Practice makes perfect:** Conduct periodic drills to familiarize everyone with the plan and refine its execution. Even if it feels silly, having perfected systems in place for everyone to understand is better than having regrets down the road.

Building an Ark of Essentials: The Emergency Supply Kit

When disaster strikes, access to resources may be limited. An emergency supply kit ensures you have the essentials to weather the storm:

- **Food and water:** Pack non-perishable food items and

bottled water sufficient for at least three days per person. Include a manual can opener and utensils. Remember to check expiration dates on products periodically to maintain freshness.

- **First-aid kit:** We covered this in an earlier chapter, but it's an excellent reminder to stock essential bandages, gauze, antiseptic wipes, pain relievers, and any prescription medications needed.
- **Flashlight and batteries:** Ensure multiple light sources are available in case of power outages. Do not store the batteries in the devices, or they may slowly drain before their use.
- **Battery-powered radio:** Stay informed about weather updates and emergency instructions. Radios with crank-capable charging for other devices, such as phones, are even better.
- **Cash and important documents:** Keep copies of passports, IDs, insurance papers, and bank statements easily accessible.
- **Personal hygiene items:** Include soap, toothbrush, toothpaste, and sanitary supplies.
- **Pet supplies:** Don't forget food, water, and bedding for your furry companions.
- **Entertainment options:** Books, cards, or battery-powered devices can help manage stress and boredom during prolonged emergencies.

Knowing When to Flee: The Decision to Evacuate

Knowing when to leave your home can be a difficult decision. Closely monitor weather warnings and emergency instructions issued by local authorities. Remember, it's always better to err on the side of caution:

- **Evacuate immediately if ordered by official authorities.**
- **Leave if floodwaters threaten your home or rising river**

levels pose a danger.
- **Don't wait until the last minute, especially if you have mobility limitations or depend on others.**

Beyond the Storm: Rebuilding and Recovery

Once the immediate danger has passed, the road to recovery begins. Remember:

- **Stay informed:** Follow official updates and instructions for safe re-entry into your neighborhood.
- **Check for damage:** Before entering, assess your home for structural damage, gas leaks, or electrical hazards.
- **Document damage:** Take photographs and videos of any damage for insurance purposes.
- **Seek help:** Don't hesitate to reach out to emergency services, relief organizations, or family and friends for assistance.

Emergency preparedness is not a one-time action, but an ongoing process. By constantly reviewing and updating your plan, maintaining your emergency kit, and staying informed about potential threats, you can transform your home into a bastion of resilience, ready to weather any storm life throws your way. Remember, the power to face the unexpected lies in preparation, knowledge, and a sense of community.

I hope this chapter empowers you to navigate the uncertain tides of natural disasters with confidence and preparedness. If you have more questions about specific types of disasters, I would suggest researching the topic further to ensure you are prepared for situations more relevant to your conditions.

CHAPTER 11: SPECIAL CONSIDERATIONS, TAILORING FIRST AID TO DIVERSE NEEDS

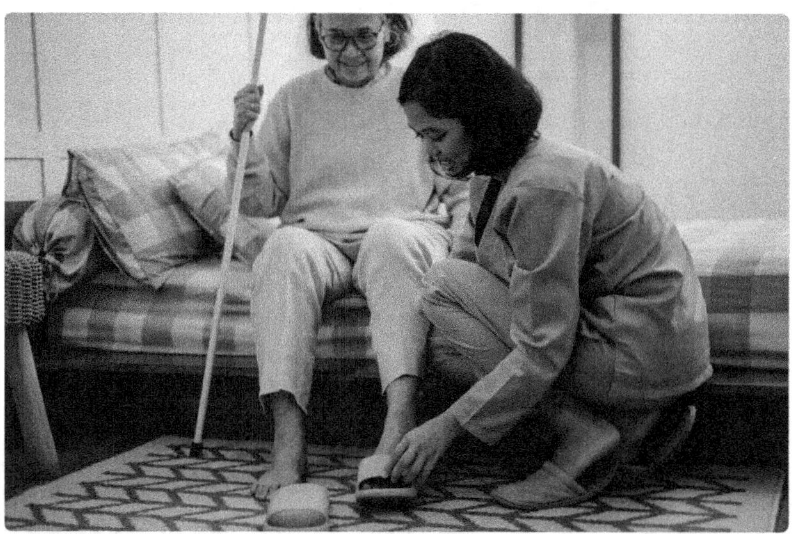

While the core principles of first aid remain constant, applying them to different individuals requires sensitivity and adjustments. This chapter delves into the unique needs of specific groups, ensuring you're equipped to handle emergencies with confidence and care, no matter who needs your help.

Fever:

A familiar enemy, yet often cloaked in confusion. We associate it with illness, discomfort, and the dreaded thermometer readings. But beneath this fiery symptom lies a fascinating story of your body's valiant fight against invaders. Let's demystify fever, understand its purpose, and learn how to handle its fiery presence with wisdom and care.

Imagine your body's internal thermostat cranked up a notch. That's essentially what happens during a fever. Your immune system, the tireless guardian, detects threats like viruses or bacteria. To combat these invaders, it releases chemicals called pyrogens, which act like messengers to the brain's "hypothalamus," the body's central temperature control center. This prompts the hypothalamus to raise the body's set point, pushing up your internal temperature – voila, a fever is born.

Why the Heat Wave?

This intentional rise in temperature is no random act of desperation. It's a strategic weapon in the immune system's arsenal. Fever has several superpowers:

- **Enzymes On Hold:** Many viruses and bacteria thrive at normal body temperatures (98.6 degrees Fahrenheit or 37 degrees Celsius is average, but people tend to run hotter or colder depending on various factors). By turning up the heat, the body slows down their growth and replication, hindering their ability to spread.
- **Defense Boost:** Fever stimulates the production of white blood cells and other immune system warriors, strengthening the body's overall defense force.
- **Protein Powerhouse:** Heat enhances the activity of specific proteins crucial for fighting infection and repairing damage.

Reading the Fire Signs:

Not all fevers are created equal. While a mild fever can

be a sign of your body doing its job, higher temperatures or those accompanied by specific symptoms might require an intervention. Here's a guide to deciphering the messages your fever might be sending:

- **Mild Fever (100-101°F):** Usually nothing to worry about, especially if accompanied by mild discomfort. Monitor the temperature and symptoms, seeking medical advice if they worsen.
- **Moderate Fever (102-103°F):** Requires closer attention, especially in infants, young children, and individuals with weakened immune systems. Consult a doctor if the fever persists for more than 24 hours with treatment, or is accompanied by worrying symptoms like severe headache, rash, difficulty breathing, or confusion.
- **High Fever (104°F or above):** Requires immediate medical attention. This can indicate a serious infection and merits prompt evaluation by a healthcare professional.

While a fever in a child can trigger worry, remember that temperature readings alone don't tell the whole story. Here's a helpful guide to deciphering the message your child's fever might be sending:

- **Mild Fever (100-101°F):** Often associated with mild discomfort and fussiness. Keep your child hydrated, ensure plenty of rest, and monitor the temperature. Seek medical advice if it persists for more than 3 days or worsens.
- **Moderate Fever (102-103°F):** Requires closer attention, especially in infants and young children. Look for accompanying symptoms like persistent crying, earache, difficulty breathing, or lethargy. Consult a pediatrician at this point on the next steps.
- **High Fever (104°F or above):** Seek immediate medical attention. This can indicate a serious infection requiring

prompt evaluation and treatment.

Beyond the Numbers: Additional Clues

While the thermometer offers valuable insights, remember to observe your child's overall behavior and well-being. Be alert for additional clues that might warrant medical attention:

- **Lethargy or excessive sleepiness:** Unusual drowsiness or difficulty staying awake can be concerning.
- **Irritability or inconsolable crying:** Excessive fussiness or persistent crying that cannot be soothed might indicate discomfort or underlying illness.
- **Loss of appetite or dehydration:** Refusal to eat or drink or signs of dehydration like dry mouth and decreased urination require medical attention.
- **Rash or skin changes:** A new rash, especially with fever, can be a symptom of certain infections and needs evaluation.
- **Difficulty breathing or chest pain:** Any signs of respiratory distress, like rapid breathing or labored breaths, demand immediate medical attention.

Cooling the Flames:

While medication can temporarily reduce fever, remember, it's just a symptom, not the disease itself. Focus on treating the underlying cause and supporting your body's natural fight. Here are some gentle ways to ease fever discomfort:

- **Hydration is Key:** Drink plenty of fluids to prevent dehydration, which is especially important during a fever. Choose water, broths, or electrolyte-rich drinks.
- **Dress Lightly:** Keep clothing loose and breathable to allow for heat dissipation.
- **Cooling Baths or Sponges:** Lukewarm baths or cool compresses applied to the forehead and wrists can provide temporary relief. Avoid using cold water or alcohol rubs, which can be counterproductive.

- **Rest and Recuperation:** Prioritize sleep and relaxation to allow your body to focus its energy on fighting the infection.
- **Medication:** Fever-reducing medication is also a great way to help reduce fever symptoms if they become overwhelming (aches and pains, higher levels, etc.). Acetaminophen, Ibuprofen, and Naproxen are common medications adults may take for a persistent fever. Never give aspirin to children, and always consult a pediatrician before giving medications to children.

Fever, though uncomfortable, is often a sign of your body's natural efforts to restore health. You can become a partner in your healing journey by understanding its purpose, reading its signals, and implementing supportive measures. Remember, seek medical advice if the fever persists or is accompanied by concerning symptoms. Together, with knowledge and care, you can navigate the fiery waves of fever and emerge stronger on the other side.

The Tiny Wonders: First Aid for Infants and Children

Little bodies require a delicate touch. Here are some key points to remember when administering first aid to infants and children:

- **Dosage matters:** Always use age-appropriate medication dosages and consult a doctor or pharmacist for guidance.
- **Calmness is key:** Children feed off your emotions. Stay calm and reassuring to minimize their distress.
- **Seek professional help promptly:** Don't hesitate to seek medical attention for even seemingly minor injuries in infants and young children.

Common childhood emergencies:

- **Fever:** Cool sponging, removing layers of clothing, and offering fluids can help manage fever.
- **Cuts and scrapes:** Clean the wound gently with sterile water, apply gentle pressure to stop bleeding, and cover

with a bandage.

- **Insect bites and stings:** Apply a cold compress to reduce swelling and use calamine lotion for itch relief. Seek medical attention for allergic reactions.
- **Seizures:** Remain calm, protect the child from harm, and time the seizure duration. Call emergency services immediately. Remove all restrictive clothing (head and neck area) and objects that could cause harm during the child's convulsing. If you can time the seizure and how many take place, it will significantly help emergency services.

The Wisdom of Age: First Aid for Elderly Individuals

The aging body presents unique challenges. Here are some considerations for first aid with seniors:

- **Chronic conditions:** Be aware of existing medical conditions and medications to avoid interactions.
- **Mobility limitations:** Adapt first aid techniques to accommodate limitations in movement.
- **Sensory decline:** Speak clearly and loudly, ensure adequate lighting, and be patient with communication.

Common senior emergencies:

- **Falls:** Check for injuries, provide support, and call emergency services if necessary.
- **Chest pain:** Seek immediate medical attention for suspected heart attack or stroke.
- **Confusion and disorientation:** Remain calm, reassure the person, and contact family or medical professionals.
- **Medication errors:** Double-check medications before administering to avoid accidental overdoses or interactions.

The Gift of Life: First Aid for Pregnant Women

Pregnancy adds another layer to the first aid equation. Here's what to remember when assisting a pregnant woman:

- **Prioritize the baby:** Always consider the potential impact on the developing fetus during any injury or medical condition.
- **Seek professional guidance:** Consult a doctor or midwife for even minor injuries or illnesses.
- **Modify techniques:** Adapt certain first aid practices to accommodate the changing body shape and potential limitations.

Common pregnancy-related emergencies:

- **Bleeding:** Seek immediate medical attention for any vaginal bleeding.
- **Abdominal pain:** Contact your doctor or midwife for any significant abdominal pain.
- **Falls:** Assess for injuries to both mother and baby, and seek medical attention if needed.
- **Fainting:** Lay the woman on her back with her legs elevated and call for help (this will redirect blood back towards the brain).

Remember: This chapter is not a substitute for professional medical advice. Always seek qualified medical assistance for any serious injury or illness, regardless of the individual's age or condition.

By understanding the unique needs of these diverse groups, you can extend your first-aid knowledge and become a confident caregiver for everyone around you. Remember, compassion, awareness, and timely action are the cornerstones of effective first aid, empowering you to make a difference in any emergency situation.

CHAPTER 12: ADDITIONAL RESOURCES AND CONCLUSION

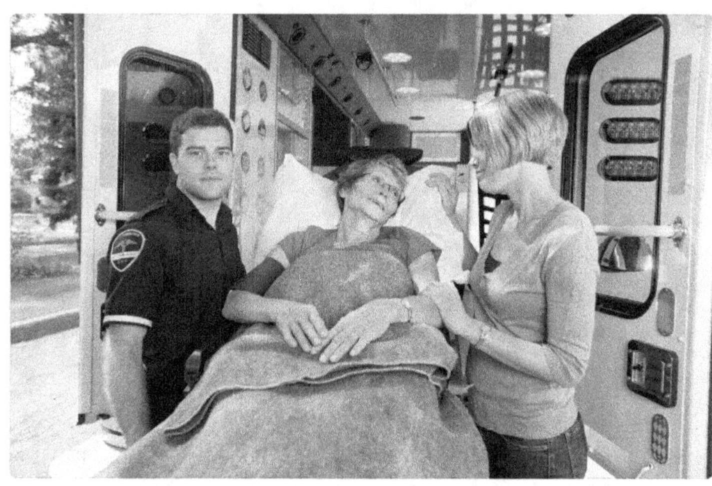

By jumping into the intricacies of first aid, you've taken a crucial step toward becoming a prepared and capable caregiver. However, the journey to lifelong learning and preparedness never ends. This chapter equips you with valuable resources to further hone your skills, stay updated on best practices, and connect with a community of first-aid enthusiasts.

Reputable Sources for First Aid Education:

- **American Red Cross:** https://www.redcross.org/take-a-class/classes/adult-first-aid%2Fcpr%2Faed-online/a6R3o000001vqDD.html Offers comprehensive online and in-person first aid training courses, including CPR and AED certification.
- **National Safety Council:** https://www.nsc.org/safety-training/first-aid/first-aid-cpr-and-aed-courses Provides various first-aid training programs, resources, and safety tips.
- **St. John Ambulance:** https://www.sja.org.uk/ A leading first aid training provider in the UK with online and in-person courses and resources.
- **Mayo Clinic:** https://www.mayoclinic.org/first-aid Offers informative articles and tips on various first-aid topics.
- **WebMD:** https://www.webmd.com/first-aid/default.htm Provides comprehensive and user-friendly information on first-aid techniques and emergencies.

Organizations and Apps for Support:

- **National Poison Control Center:** https://poisonhelp.hrsa.gov/poison-centers/find-poison-center Provides 24/7 access to poison specialists in case of accidental ingestions or overdoses.
- **Stop the Bleed:** https://www.stopthebleed.org/find-a-course/ Empowers individuals to learn basic bleeding control techniques in emergency situations.
- **American Trauma Care Association:** https://www.amtrauma.org/ Offers resources and education on trauma care and emergency preparedness.
- **First Aid Responder App:** https://play.google.com/store/apps/details?id=au.com.stjohnambulance.stjohnappprod&hl=en_AU Provides step-by-step instructions for various first-aid scenarios and medical emergencies.

Conclusion:

The knowledge and skills acquired through this journey equip you to navigate the unpredictable waters of emergencies with confidence and resilience. Remember, first aid is not just about mastering techniques; it's about fostering a mindset of preparedness, a willingness to step forward, and a dedication to making a difference when those around you need it most.

Continue nurturing your first-aid knowledge, explore the resources provided, and share your skills with others. By building a community of empowered individuals, we can weave a safety net, ensuring that the knowledge and confidence to help are always within reach wherever life's journeys may lead.

Congratulations on completing this journey towards first-aid preparedness! Remember, this is just the beginning, and the road to mastering lifesaving skills is one of continuous learning and growth. Embrace the journey, stay informed, and always be ready to lend a helping hand. Together, we can create a world where everyone has the potential to be a lifesaver.

Feel free to return for any further inquiries, clarifications, or discussions on specific topics you encountered throughout this journey. I am here to assist you in expanding your knowledge and refining your skills as you navigate the ever-evolving landscape of first aid.

www.ingramcontent.com/pod-product-compliance
Lightning Source LLC
Chambersburg PA
CBHW061002260726
48661CB00005B/2016